Published By Adam Gilbin

@ Daniel Marsh

I0096747

The Carnivore Diet Cookbook: The Most Simple

Diet for Meat Lovers to Burn Fat Fast and 160+

Delicious Carnivorous Recipes

ISBN 978-1-990666-84-1

TABLE OF CONTENTS

Fish Tacos With Avocado Crema Recipe

Ingredients:

- Avocado crema sauce, 3 tablespoon

- Chopped avocado, 2

- Chopped cilantro, a bunch

- Salsa,2 cup

- Chopped red onion, 1

- Chicken fish filet, 2 pound

- Olive oil, 6 tablespoon

- Taco shells, 9

- Salt and pepper to taste

Directions:

1. Add the olive oil, salt, and pepper to the fish filet.
2. Grill the filet for ten minutes and then slice it up.
3. Heat the taco shells and start filling them with fish slices, avocado crema sauce, red onions, salsa, avocado slices and cilantro on top.
4. Your dish is ready to be served.

Garlic Butter Prawns Recipe

Ingredients:

- Minced garlic, 3 tablespoon

- Minced ginger, 2 tablespoon

- Lemon juice, 1 cup

- Butter, 2 tablespoon

- Fresh herbs, 2 tablespoon

- Mix spice, 2 teaspoon

- Onion, 2 cup

- Prawn pieces, 1 pound

- Smoked paprika, 1 teaspoon

- Chopped cilantro, as required

- Chopped tomatoes, 2 cup

Directions:

1. Take a pan. Add in the butter and onions.
2. Cook the onions until they become soft and fragrant.
3. Add in the chopped garlic and ginger.
4. Cook the mixture and add the tomatoes into it.
5. Add the spices and fresh herbs.
6. When the tomatoes are d2, add the prawn pieces into it.
7. Mix the Ingredients: carefully and place your mixture into the oven.
8. When your prawns are d2, dish them out.
9. Add fresh herbs on top.
10. Your dish is ready to be served.

Seas2d Tilapia Fillets

Ingredients:

- ¼ teaspoon of paprika

- ¼ teaspoon of dried thyme

- 1/8 teaspoon of onion powder

- 1/8 teaspoon of salt

- 1/8 teaspoon of pepper

- 2 tilapia fillets (6 ounces each)

- 1 tablespoon of melted butter

- 1 teaspoon of steak seasoning

- ½ teaspoon of dried parsley flakes

- A dash of garlic powder

Directions:

1. Preheat oven to 425 degrees F and place the tilapia in a greased baking pan then, drizzle it with butter.
2. In a small bowl, mix the remaining Ingredients: and sprinkle over the fillets.
3. Bake it covered for 10 minutes.
4. Uncover it then, bake until the fish just begins to flake easily.

Steamed Lobster

Ingredients:

- 4 lobster tails

- 125g butter, melted

- Tablespoon sea salt

Directions:

1. Fill a large pot with about 1 inch of water and bring to the boil.
2. Add the salt and place a steamer insert inside the pot so that it is just above the water level.
3. Place the lobster tails inside the steamer and cover the pot.
4. Steam them for at most 8 minutes without taking off the lid.
5. Serve with melted butter.

Chicken And Bacon Sausages

Ingredients:

- 2 tsp onion powder

- ½ tsp salt

- ½ tsp pepper

- 1 lb chicken breasts

- 2 slices bacon, cooked, crumbled

- 1 egg, whisked

- 2 tbsp Italian seasoning

- 2 tsp garlic powder

Directions:

1. Preheat the oven to 425° F.
2. Put all the Ingredients: into a food processor and process well.

3. From the meat mixture form approximately 12 thin patties (½-inch thick) and place on a baking tray lined with foil.
4. Bake for 20 minutes, until a meat thermometer shows 170° F.
5. Serve immediately or store in the freezer for 4 weeks.

Whole Roast Chicken

Ingredients:

- 2 garlic cloves

- 1 tsp Herbes de Provence

- 1 tbsp coarse sea salt

- 3 lbs whole organic chicken

- 2 sprigs fresh rosemary

Directions:

1. Preheat oven to 350°F.
2. Rinse the chicken well under cold water.
3. Place chicken on a baking pan, breast up.
4. Stuff the cavity with the garlic cloves and rosemary.
5. Mix the salt and Herbes the Provence in a small bowl. Sprinkle 1 of the mixture on the breast.

6. Turn chicken breast side down and sprinkle the remaining mixture on the top.
7. Bake for 1 hour 30 minutes, until the chicken skin is nicely browned.
8. Serve immediately.

Beef Kabobs

Ingredients:

- 2 teaspoons fresh thyme, minced

- 4 tablespoons butter, melted

- 2 tablespoons fresh lemon juice

- Salt and freshly ground black pepper, to taste

- 2 pounds beef sirloin, cut into cubes

- 3 garlic cloves, minced

- 1 tablespoon fresh lemon zest, grated

- 2 teaspoons fresh rosemary, minced

- 2 teaspoons fresh parsley, minced

- 2 teaspoons fresh oregano, minced

Directions:

1. In a bowl, add all the Ingredients: except the beef and mix well.

2. Add the beef and coat with the herb mixture generously.

3. Refrigerate to marinate for at least 20-30 minutes.

4. Preheat the grill to medium-high heat. Grease the grill grate.

5. Remove the beef cubes from the marinade and thread onto metal skewers.

6. Place the skewers onto the grill and cook for about 6-8 minutes, flipping after every 2 minutes.

7. Remove from the grill and place onto a platter for about 5 minutes before serving.

Shrimp Kabobs

Ingredients:

- 1 garlic cloves, minced

- ½ teaspoon paprika

- Salt and freshly ground black pepper, to taste

- 1 pound medium raw shrimp, peeled and deveined

- ¼ cup butter, melted

- 2 tablespoons fresh lime juice

Directions:

1. Ina large bowl, add the butter, lime juice, garlic, paprika, salt and black pepper and mix well.

2. Add the shrimp and coat with the garlic mixture generously.

3. Refrigerate to marinate for at least 30 minutes.

4. Preheat the grill to medium-high heat. Grease the grill grate.

5. Thread the shrimp onto the pre-soaked wooden skewers.

6. Place the skewers onto the grill and cook for about 2-4 minutes per side.

7. Remove from the grill and place the shrimp kabobs onto a platter for about 5 minutes before serving.

Grilled Chicken Breasts

Ingredients:

- 3 tablespoons fresh parsley, chopped

- 3 tablespoons butter, melted

- 3 tablespoons fresh lemon juice

- 1 teaspoon paprika

- ½ teaspoon dried oregano

- 4 (4-ounce) b2less, skinless chicken breast halves

- 3 garlic cloves, chopped finely

- Salt and freshly ground black pepper, to taste

Directions:

1. With a fork, pierce chicken breasts several times.

2. In a large bowl, add all the Ingredients: except the chicken breasts and mix until well combined.
3. Add the chicken breasts and coat with the marinade generously.
4. Refrigerate to marinate for about 2-3 hours.
5. Preheat the grill to medium-high heat. Grease the grill grate.
6. Remove the chicken from the bowl and shake off excess marinade.
7. Place the chicken breasts onto the grill and cook for about 5-6 minutes per side.
8. Remove from the grill and transfer the chicken breasts onto the serving plate.
9. Serve hot alongside the yogurt sauce.

Instant Pot Chicken Bone Broth

Ingredients:

- 5 cloves garlic, whole

- 1 tomato, roughly chopped

- 6 black peppercorns

- 1 teaspoon apple cider vinegar

- ½ teaspoon salt, or to taste

- 1 chicken carcass

- 2 medium onions, roughly chopped

- 2 medium carrots, roughly chopped

- 2 stalks celery, leaves included, coarsely chopped

- water

Directions:

1. Preheat the oven to 350 degrees F (175 degrees C). Line a baking pan with aluminum foil.

2. Place chicken carcass, onions, carrots, celery, and garlic on the prepared baking pan.

3. Bake in the preheated oven until carcass is browned, about 1 hour.

4. Remove pan from oven; scrape carcass and roasted vegetables into an electric pressure cooker. Add tomato, peppercorns, cider vinegar, and salt. Fill pot 2/3 full with water; close and lock the lid. Select the Soup setting according to manufacturer's instructions and set timer for 30 minutes. Allow 10 to 15 minutes for pressure to build.

5. Release pressure using the natural-release method according to manufacturer's instructions, 10 to 40 minutes.

6. Strain broth through a layer of cheesecloth into another container. Let cool, at least 20 minutes. Cover and refrigerate until a layer of fat solidifies on the surface, 4 hours to overnight. Remove and discard the fat.

Cajun Shrimp

Ingredients:

- ¼ teaspoon salt

- ¼ teaspoon ground black pepper

- ¼ teaspoon cayenne pepper, or more to taste

- 1 ½ pounds large shrimp, peeled and deveined

- 1 tablespoon vegetable oil

- 1 teaspoon paprika

- ¾ teaspoon dried thyme

- ¾ teaspoon dried oregano

- ¼ teaspoon garlic powder

Directions:

1. Combine paprika, thyme, oregano, garlic powder, salt, pepper, and cayenne pepper in a sealable plastic bag; shake to mix.
2. Add shrimp and shake to coat.
3. Heat oil in a large non-stick skillet over medium high heat.
4. Cook and stir shrimp in hot oil until they are bright pink on the outside and the meat is no longer transparent in the center, about 4 minutes.

Lamb Chops For The Grill

Ingredients:

- 1 tbsp fresh rosemary (finely chopped)

- 3 cloves garlic (minced)

- ½ tsp sea salt

- 8 lamb chops (about ¾ inch thickness)

- 3 tbsp extra virgin olive oil

- Freshly ground black pepper to taste

Directions:

1. Preheat the grill or stove top grill pan to a medium-high heat.

2. Mix all the marinade Ingredients: together in a small mixing bowl. Spread this mixture evenly over all sides of the lamb chops.

3. Grill the lamb chops for 2 to 4 minutes on each side until they are tender (135°F for medium rare). Transfer the chops to a serving platter and let them rest for 6-10 minutes before serving.

Crispy Beef Liver

Ingredients:

- 1 tbsp fresh mint (chopped)

- 1 tsp sea salt

- ¼ tsp black pepper freshly ground

- 1 lb beef liver (cut into thin slices)

- ½ cup olive oil

- 1 clove garlic (crushed)

Directions:

1. Preheat a large grill pan over medium-high heat.
2. Rinse the liver under cold running water.
3. Make sure to rinse out all of the blood. Pat it dry with a paper towel.

4. Using a sharp knife, remove the rough veins, if there are any. Cut it crossways into thin slices.

5. In a small mixing bowl, combine the olive oil with the crushed garlic, mint, salt, and pepper.

6. Mix until everything is well combined. Brush the liver slices with this mixture and grill for 5-7 minutes on each side.

7. Serve immediately for the best results.

Easy Seafood Stock

Ingredients:

- 1 leek, white and pale green part only (thinly sliced)

- 1 stalk celery (chopped)

- 6 peppercorns

- 4-½ cups cold water

- 4 oz shrimp shells (from about 15-20 shrimp)

- 1 tsp soybean oil

- ¾ cup onion (chopped)

Directions:

1. Warm-up a stockpot or a large saucepan.
2. To start, add some oil to a hot pan.
3. Then, add some shrimp shells to the hot oil.

4. Sauté the pellets until they are bright pink or reddish in color, then remove them from the pan.

5. Add the vegetables and stir them together. It's time to turn the heat down and let it sweat for about 3 minutes.

6. Add the spices and water, then turn the heat up to high.

7. Bring the stock to a boil, lower the heat and let it simmer for about 20 to 25 minutes, until it's thick.

8. Set it aside and let it cool down a little. It's then time to strain the stock through a strainer with a fine mesh inside it.

9. Add it to a container of your choice and store it in the fridge or freezer until ready to use it.

Slow Cooker Carnivore Beef Stew

Ingredients:

- 6 cups b2 broth

- 8 oz mushrooms (quartered)

- 1 large onion chopped

- 4 cloves garlic minced

- 2 tsp dried thyme

- 2 tsp salt

- 2 lb beef marrow b2s

- 2 lb chuck roast cubed

- 2 tbsp beef tallow

- 1 tsp ground black pepper

Directions:

1. Make sure the slow cooker is on a low setting.

2. Place the marrow b2s in the middle and close the lid.

3. In a large skillet, heat up the tallow over high heat.

4. Cube the roast and put it in the skillet. When you put the meat on the pan, cook it on all sides.

5. When the heart is d2, put it in the pot.

6. Rinse and chop all vegetables, gather the herbs, and put them in the pot with the meat.

7. Pour the broth over the Ingredients:, season them with salt and pepper, and then serve.

8. Cook on low for 6-8 hours. Then, put it away and let it cool down.

9. Then, put it in freezer-friendly containers.

10. To enjoy: Freeze the food in separate containers and heat it up when you are ready to eat it in the oven or microwave.

Quick And Easy Egg Drop Soup

Ingredients:

- 1/2 teaspoon ginger powder

- 1/2 teaspoon coconut aminos

- 1/8 teaspoon ground black pepper

- 1/4 teaspoon salt

- 2 cups b2 broth (lamb, goat, chicken, or beef)

- 3 whole eggs whisked

- Red chili pepper flakes optional

Directions:

1. Warm broth in a small saucepan over medium heat.

2. Whisk eggs in a bowl. Add ginger powder and mix well.

3. Once little bubbles begin to rise in the broth, just before boiling, stir in a circular motion and slowly pour in the whisked eggs.
4. Leave to cook for one minute, or until eggs are done to your liking.
5. Pour into a serving bowl, season with coconut aminos, salt and pepper and the optional chili flakes. Taste and adjust as needed.

Keto Carnivore Braised Beef Shank + Oven, Crockpot, & Instant Pot Option

Ingredients:

- 2-3 cups Carnivore Diet Bone Broth or water

- 1 teaspoon salt plus extra as needed

- 1 tablespoon beef tallow butter, ghee, or other cooking fat

- 4 pieces beef shank 1-inch thick, 8 ounces each

Directions:

1. Heat cooking fat in a cast iron or heavy bottom skillet with a lid or Dutch oven.

2. Brown both sides of the beef shanks, about 2-3 minutes per side, until a golden-brown crust forms.

3. Pour broth over shanks. Use at least 2 cups of broth.

4. There should be enough broth to cover the meat ½ to ¾ of the way up the side.

5. Season with salt. Bring it to a simmer.

6. Reduce the heat and cover with a lid, but leave a small opening for the steam to escape.

7. Cook over low heat for 3 hours, until the meat falls off the bone. Serve warm in liquid.

Keto Eggnog Pudding

Ingredients:

- 1 cup water

- 1 teaspoon ground cinnamon

- 1 teaspoon ground nutmeg

- 20 drops Liquid monkfruit sweetener

- 1 tablespoon grass-fed beef gelatin

- 1.5 cups heavy whipping cream

Directions:

1. Sprinkle gelatin over the cream. Leave this aside to "bloom" or sit and thicken.

2. Bring the water to a simmer on the stove. Remove from heat, whisk in the cinnamon, nutmeg and Lakanto sweetener.

3. Add the thickened cream to the saucepan and mix well until all gelatin dissolves.

4. Pour into individual pudding cups (ramekins) or one main serving dish.

5. Refrigerate for one hour or until completely set. Serve chilled.

Soup With Cheddar Chicken

Ingredients:

- 2 cups cheddar cheese, shredded

- 6 quarts chicken stock

- to taste salt

- 1 teaspoon of butter

- 1 pound skinless, b2less chicken breasts, sliced into bite-size portions

- 4 quarts milk

Directions:

1. Place a medium saucepan over medium heat. Melt the butter in the pan.

2. Add the chicken and cook for a few minutes, or until it is nicely coated with butter.

3. Combine the broth and milk in a mixing bowl. Cook until the chicken is cooked through.

4. Turn the heat off.

5. Stir in the cheese and salt until the cheese has melted.

6. Serve immediately in soup bowls.

Turkey With Salt And Pepper.

Ingredients:

- butter (3-5 tablespoons)

- to taste coarse salt

- to taste freshly ground pepper

- 1 whole turkey (9-10 pounds), giblets removed

Directions:

1. In a large roasting pan, pour 2 cups of water. In the pan, place a rack.

2. Start with the neck and work your way up to the breasts. Take a little amount of the butter and massage it into your skin.

3. Season the turkey and the cavity well with salt and pepper. Tie the legs together with a strong kitchen thread. Tuck the turkey wings underneath the bird on the rack.

4. Bake for 2-3 hours at 350 degrees F, or until an instant read thermometer in the thickest part of the meat registers 165 degrees F.

5. After every 25 to 30 minutes, baste the turkey with the remaining butter. Shake the turkey gently to release the cooked juices into the pan.

6. Place the turkey on a chopping board after removing it from the oven. Allow 30 minutes after covering with foil.

7. Cut into slices when cool enough to handle. Serve with some of the pan's cooking liquid drizzled over the turkey.

Cream Sauced Turkey

Ingredients:

- 34 cup chicken stock, pepper to taste

- 2 cups cooked turkey, chopped

- 3 tbsp. melted butter

- a quarter-cup of heavy cream

- to taste salt

Directions:

1. Preheat a large skillet over medium-high heat. Cook the butter until it gets golden brown.

2. Simmer for 5-6 minutes after adding the stock.

3. Cream, turkey, salt, and pepper to taste. Cook for a couple of minutes.

4. Serve immediately.

Beef Casserole

Ingredients:

- 1 small Anaheim pepper, seeded and roughly chopped

- ½ red bell pepper, seeded and roughly chopped

- 6 white mushrooms, trimmed and halved

- 1 anchovy, minced

- 1 tablespoon minced garlic

- 1 tablespoon soy sauce

- 1 tablespoon balsamic vinegar

- 1 tablespoon Worcestershire sauce

- 2 tablespoons tomato paste

- 2 tablespoons olive oil

- 5 cups beef broth, divided, plus

- ½ cup if needed

- ½ medium leek, trimmed, and thinly sliced

- ½ onion, thinly sliced

- 2 medium celery stalks, roughly chopped

- 1 teaspoon beef bouillon powder

Directions:

1. Preheat the oven to 325°F.

2. A small bowl should have the salt, paprika, and black pepper. Mix them and put them in the small bowl. It helps to pat the meat dry with paper towels. Then, rub the salt mixture on both sides of the essence and dry it.

3. When the olive oil is hot, put it in a Dutch oven. This is how it should look when the

steak is d2 cooking: Set it on a plate and put it away. Heat is off.

4. It's time to add 12 cups of beef broth to the Dutch oven. Let it heat up until it bubbles and spits a lot. Deglaze the Dutch oven with a spatula. Scrape up any brown bits from the pan with the tool.

5. Turn down the heat to medium-high, then add the leek and onion and celery and bell pepper and mushrooms and anchovies and garlic and soy sauce and balsamic vinegar and Worcestershire sauce and tomato paste, and stir until everything is mixed.

6. Add the remaining 4 12 cups of beef broth and the bouillon powder and cook, stirring, until it comes to a gentle boil.

7. It's time to cover the Dutch oven, put it in the oven, and bake for 3 hours. Check the liquid to see if it's low, then see if it is. Then add another 12 cups of broth.

8. Bake for another hour. Cover the meat in the Dutch oven and let it rest for 30 minutes before you serve it. TIP: The long, slow cooking at a low temperature makes the meat soft and juicy.

9. If you want to cook it faster, don't do it on a higher heat. The heart will be hard.

Perfect Pork Chops

Ingredients:

- 2 teaspoons freshly ground black pepper

- 4 garlic cloves, peeled

- ½ small onion, thinly sliced

- 6 mushrooms, quartered (optional; see Tip)

- 1 sprig fresh rosemary

- 2 tablespoons olive oil

- 2 (11-ounce) b2-in pork chops

- 2 teaspoons kosher salt

- 2 tablespoons salted butter

Directions:

1. Preheat the oven to 400°F.

2. Heat the olive oil in a small, cast-iron pan over high heat for 5 minutes.

3. Salt and pepper both sides of the pork chops.

4. Make sure you don't move the pork chops in the skillet while cooking.

5. Add the garlic, onion, and mushrooms to the chops and spread them out around them, then cook.

6. Turn the chops over, put the rosemary sprig on top, add the butter to the skillet, then stir it all together.

7. Take care when you put the skillet in the oven.

8. Roast the pork chops for 8 minutes, or until the internal temperature is between 145°F and 155°F, then serve.

9. Before you eat: Take out of the oven, cover the skillet with aluminum foil, and let it rest for about 5 minutes before you serve it. TIP:

10. To make this a C4 dish, you can leave the mushrooms and onions and still have it.

Brown Sugar Glazed Salmon Recipe

Ingredients:

- Salmon pieces, 1 pound

- Chopped cilantro, as required

- Minced garlic, 3 tablespoon

- Minced ginger, 3 tablespoon

- Brown sugar, 1 cup

- Butter, 3 tablespoon

- Fresh herbs, 2 tablespoon

- Chopped tomatoes, 2 cup

Directions:

1. Take a pan.

2. Add the chopped garlic and ginger.

3. Cook the mixture and add the tomatoes into it.

4. Add the fresh herbs.

5. Add the salmon pieces into it.

6. Mix the Ingredients: carefully and add the brown sugar on top of the salmon pieces.

7. Place your mixture into the oven.

8. When salmons are d2, dish them out.

9. Your dish is ready to be served.

Slow Cooker Fish And Tomatoes Recipe

Ingredients:

- Mix spices, 3 tablespoon

- Minced garlic, 3 tablespoon

- Minced ginger, 3 tablespoon

- Cilantro, 1 cup

- Olive oil, 3 tablespoon

- Cherry tomatoes, 3 cup

- Vegetable broth, 2 cup

- Onion, 2 cup

- B2less fish, 3 cups

- Smoked paprika, 1 teaspoon

- Water, 2 cup

Directions:

1. Take a pan.
2. Add in the oil and onions.
3. Cook the onions until they become soft and fragrant.
4. Add in the chopped garlic and ginger.
5. Cook the mixture and add the tomatoes into it.
6. Add in the broth, fish and spices.
7. Mix the Ingredients: carefully and cover your pan.
8. Mix your dish and let it cook for an additional forty-five minutes.
9. Add cilantro on top.
10. Your dish is ready to be served.

Liver With Lemon Thyme

Ingredients:

- 10 sprigs fresh lemon thyme, chopped

- Salt and pepper to taste

- Lb. calves liver

- Tablespoon olive oil

Directions:

1. First, rinse the liver and pat dry.
2. Then, with a sharp knife, remove any exposed veins, ducts or connective tissue.
3. Next, use your fingers to remove the thin outer membrane, being careful not to tear the liver itself.
4. From there, slice the liver into about ¼ inch thick slices.
5. Rinse again and pat dry. Next, heat olive oil in a large pot over medium heat.

6. Add the fresh thyme to the pan, and then lay the liver on top.

7. Cook over medium heat for about 4 minutes, then flip and cook on other side the liver should be eaten slightly pink, so take care not to overcook as it can make the liver tough.

8. Season it with salt and pepper as

Duck Leg Confit

Ingredients:

- ½ tsp black pepper

- 10 garlic cloves

- 4 bay leaves

- 4 sprigs fresh thyme

- 1½ tsp black peppercorns

- 4 duck legs with thighs attached, excess duck fat trimmed and reserved

- 1 tbsp + ¼ tsp kosher salt

- ½ tsp table salt

- 4 cups olive oil

Directions:

1. Put the reserved duck fat in the bottom of a plastic or glass container.

2. On a platter, lay 3 duck legs, skin side down. Season with black pepper, 1 tbsp kosher salt, thyme, garlic cloves, and bay leaves.

3. Lay the remaining 3 duck legs on top, flesh to flesh. Sprinkle with the remaining ¼ tsp kosher salt. Cover and refrigerate for 12 hours.

4. Preheat the oven to 300°F.

5. Remove duck legs from the fridge.

6. Remove and reserve the thyme, garlic, bay leaves, and duck fat. Rinse the duck legs with cold water, rubbing off some of the pepper and salt. Pat dry with paper towels.

7. In the bottom of an enamel cast iron pot, put the reserved bay leaves, garlic, duck fat, and thyme. Sprinkle with the salt and peppercorns.

8. Lay the duck legs in the pot, skin side down, and add the olive oil.

9. Cover and bake for 2.5-3 hours, or until the meat pulls away from the b2.

10. Remove the duck from the fat. Strain the fat and reserve.

11. In a hot pan, sear duck legs skin-side down until the skin is crispy and golden, about 3-4 minutes. Serve immediately.

Turkey Meatballs

Ingredients:

- ¾ cup Parmesan cheese, grated

- 1 tbsp dried parsley

- 1¼ lb turkey, minced

- 1 tbsp dried minced onion

- 1 clove garlic, finely minced

- ¾ cup milk

- ⅓ cup crushed pork rinds

- 1 large egg

- 1 tsp salt

- ½ tsp freshly ground black pepper

Directions:

1. Combine all Ingredients: together in a large bowl.

2. Using large scoop, form mixture into even-sized balls and place on a baking sheet.

3. Preheat the oven to 400°F and bake for 25-30 minutes.

Turkey Scotch Eggs

Ingredients:

- 6 hard-boiled eggs, cooled, peeled, dry

- 1 lb ground turkey

- 1 egg

- 2 tsp garlic powder

- 1 tsp poultry seasoning

- ½ tbsp Cajun seasoning

Grain-free breading:

- ¼ cup Parmesan cheese

- ½ tsp salt

- ½ tsp black pepper

Directions:

1. Preheat the oven to 400° F.

2. In a bowl, combine the turkey, garlic powder, poultry seasoning, and Cajun seasoning. Mix well. Make 6 patties.

3. Beat an egg in a separate bowl.

4. In another bowl, mix the grain-free breading Ingredients:.

5. Place hard-boiled egg on a patty, and roll in hands around the egg until covered and ball-shaped.

6. Dip and roll in egg, then roll in cheese mixture till covered.

7. Place on a parchment-lined casserole baking dish.

8. Bake for 30 minutes. Then broil on low for 2-3 minutes, just until browned.

9. Serve immediately.

Pan-Seared Pork Chops

Ingredients:

- ½ teaspoon garlic paste

- Salt and freshly ground black pepper, to taste

- 4 (6-ounce) (½-inch thick) b2less pork chops

- 2 tablespoons butter, melted

- 1 tablespoon Worcestershire sauce

- 1 teaspoon fresh lemon juice

Directions:

1. In a large bowl, add all the Ingredients: except for pork chops and mix well.
2. Add the pork chops and coat with the mixture generously.
3. Cover the bowl and set aside at room temperature for about 10-15 minutes.

4. Heat a greased skillet over medium-high heat and cook the pork chops for about 5 minutes, gently shaking the skillet occasionally.

5. Flip the pork chops and reduce heat to low.

6. Cook for about 1-2 minutes.

7. Serve hot

Grilled Lamb Chops

Ingredients:

- 1 teaspoon garlic, minced

- Salt and freshly ground black pepper, to taste

- 4 (8-ounce) (½-inch-thick) lamb shoulder blade chops

- ¼ cup butter, melted

- 2 tablespoons fresh lemon juice

- 2 tablespoons fresh oregano, chopped

Directions:

1. In a bowl, place all Ingredients: and beat until well combined.
2. Place the chops and marinade into a large sealable plastic bag.

3. Seal the bag and shake vigorously to coat evenly.

4. Set aside at room temperature for about 1 hour.

5. Remove the lamb chops from the bag and discard the marinade.

6. With paper towels, pat dry the lamb chops.

7. Season the lamb chops with a little salt.

8. Preheat a large cast-iron grill pan over medium-high heat and cook 2 lamb chops for about 3 minutes.

9. Move the lamb chops and cook for about 3 more minutes.

10. Now, flip the lamb chops to their sides and adjust the heat to medium-low.

11. Cook for about 2-3 minutes.

12. Repeat with the remaining lamb chops.

13. Remove the lamb chops from heat and set aside for about 5 minutes before serving.

Barbecued Shrimp

Ingredients:

- 6 slices bacon, cut in half

- ¼ cup barbecue sauce

- 12 large shrimp

- 6 ounces provolone cheese, cut into 12 strips

- ¼ cup green chile peppers, diced

Directions:

1. Peel, devein and butterfly the shrimp or prawns. (To butterfly shrimp: Split shrimp down the center, cutting almost completely through.)

2. Insert a strip of provolone cheese and 1 teaspoon of the diced green chilies into each shrimp.

3. Fold over the shrimp and wrap with a 1 strip of bacon.

4. Secure with wooden picks.

5. Cook shrimp on grill, basting with your favorite barbecue sauce, until bacon is cooked and shrimp is pink.

Sauteed Shrimp

Ingredients:

- 1 sprig fresh rosemary, chopped, or to taste

- ¼ teaspoon dried basil

- ¼ teaspoon dried oregano

- ¼ teaspoon ground coriander

- 1 bay leaf

- ¾ cup white wine, or to taste

- 1 teaspoon Worcestershire sauce, or to taste

- 1 lemon

- 3 pounds uncooked medium shrimp, peeled and deveined

- 1 tablespoon olive oil

- 1 small onion, chopped

- 2 ribs celery, chopped

- 2 cloves garlic, crushed and chopped

- salt and ground black pepper to taste

Directions:

1. Squeeze lemon over shrimp and set aside.
2. Heat olive oil over medium heat. Add onion, celery, and garlic.
3. Season with salt and pepper and cook until tender, about 5 minutes.
4. Stir in rosemary, basil, oregano, coriander, and bay leaf.
5. Add white wine and Worcestershire sauce; cook until sauce is slightly reduced and flavors come together, 8 to 10 minutes.
6. Add shrimp to the sauce and cook until pink, 5 to 7 minutes more.

Roast Beef Brisket

Ingredients:

- 3 large carrots

- 1 small cabbage (chopped)

- 1 tsp bay leaf (crushed)

- 2-3 cups beef stock (homemade)

- 1 tsp mustard powder

- 4 lb beef brisket

- 2 tbsp olive oil

- 3 large onions

- 3 cloves garlic (minced)

- 3 stalks of celery

Directions:

1. The day before you plan on serving the brisket, be sure to boil it in water to cover for 2 hours and refrigerate until the next day.

2. Preheat the oven to 300°F.

3. Add olive oil to a pan and brown the brisket on all sides. Once browned, set the brisket aside.

4. Add the garlic and onion to the pan and cook until brown.

5. Put the brisket in a baking dish, add all the Ingredients:, and cover.

6. Bake it for 4 hours, turning the brisket every hour (add water if necessary).

7. You can also make gravy from the leftover stock, and be sure to cut the meat against the grain before serving.

Broiled Pram Tilapia

Ingredients:

- 1 tbsp freshly squeezed lemon juice

- ⅛ tsp dried basil

- ⅛ tsp ground black pepper

- ⅛ tsp onion powder

- ⅛ tsp celery salt

- 1 lb tilapia fillets

- ¼ cup Parmesan cheese (shredded)

- 2 tbsp unsalted butter (softened)

- 1 tbsp plus ½ tsp reduced sugar mayonnaise

Directions:

1. Preheat your oven's broiler. Grease a broiling pan or line with aluminum foil.

2. In a small mixing bowl, mix the Parmesan cheese, mayonnaise, butter, and lemon juice together.

3. Season the mixture with dried basil, onion powder, pepper, and celery salt. Mix well and set aside.

4. Place the fillets in a single layer on the prepared pan.

5. Broil the fillets a few inches away from the heat for 2-3 minutes.

6. Flip the fillets over and broil for an additional 2-3 minutes.

7. Remove the fillets from the oven and cover them with the cheese mixture on the top.

8. Broil the fillets for another 2-3 minutes or until the topping is browned and the fish flakes easily with a fork.

9. Be careful not to overcook the fish as it could become dry or tough.

10. Let it cool down completely before storing it in the fridge.

11. It is also best to let it breathe before covering it with any type of lid.

Carnivore Beef Broth

Ingredients:

- 2 tbsp organic apple cider vinegar

- 1 tsp sea salt (to taste)

- 12 garlic cloves

- 2 lb grass-fed marrow b2s

- 1 gallon filtered water

Directions:

1. Brown the marrow b2s in a greased pan to add some flavor.
2. Add all the Ingredients: into a crock pot.
3. Cook it on high until the broth starts to boil, then switch it to low and cook for an additional 10-24 hours.
4. Remember, longer is always better when it comes to broth.

5. Let the broth cool, and then transfer it to glass jars or any containers of your choice.

6. Store it in the fridge for a few days or freeze it if you would like to keep it longer.

Carnivore Steak Nuggets

Ingredients:

- ½ cup pork panko

- ½ tsp homemade seas2d salt

- Dip (optional)

- ¼ cup mayonnaise

- ¼ cup sour cream (organic, cultured)

- 1+ tsp chipotle paste to taste

- 1 lb venison or beef steak cut into chunks

- 1 large egg

- Lard or palm oil

- Breading

- ½ cup grated Parmesan cheese

- ½ tsp homemade ranch dressing and dip mix

- ¼ medium lime (juiced)

Directions:

1. For the dip: Combine all of the Ingredients: and mix it thoroughly. 1 tsp of the chipotle paste produces a medium-spice variety; use more or less according to taste. Refrigerate 30 minutes before serving and remember that it can be kept refrigerated for up to 1 week.

2. Combine the pork panko, Parmesan cheese and seas2d salt and set aside.

3. Beat 1 egg and place the beaten egg in a mixing bowl and the breading mix in another.

4. Dip the cut pieces of steak in the egg, and follow with the breading. Place it on a wax paper lined sheet pan or plate.

5. Freeze the breaded raw steak bites for 30 minutes before frying. This way, the breading will not pull away from the meat while frying.

6. Heat the lard or oil to roughly 325°F. Fry the steak nuggets (from frozen) until browned, for about 2-3 minutes.

7. Transfer to a paper towel lined dish, flavor with a sprinkle of salt, and serve it with or without the dip.

Simple Liver And Onions

Ingredients:

- ¼ cup flour (optional)

- 1 tsp black pepper

- ¼ tsp garlic powder

- 1-2 cups of water

- 1 lb calf liver

- 1 medium onion (chopped)

- 1 tbsp extra virgin olive oil

Directions:

1. Heat the oil in a pan. Then, if you want to, coat the pieces of liver in flour and put them in the pan.

2. Remove the liver from the pan and brown it on both sides.

3. Add the onions and garlic powder, cook them until they are transparent, and add the chicken.

4. Add flour, 2 tablespoon, until the oil is g2 and the flour is a little brown.

5. Add water to the flour and onion mixture until it reaches a gravy consistency that you like, then stir in the salt and pepper.

6. Let it cook for about 5 minutes, then add the liver. Do this for about 10 minutes.

7. Cover it with a lid and let it cook for another 10-15 minutes, then turn off the heat.

8. To make this recipe, you don't need to add flour. It's good even without it!

9. You can also use some finely grated Parmesan cheese instead of the flour in this recipe.

10. People who follow the carnivore diet and use flour should know that this dish should not be eaten very often because it has more

carbohydrates than is recommended for people who do.

Freezer-Friendly Italian Meatballs

Ingredients:

- 1 egg

- 2 tsp dried parsley

- 1 tsp dried Italian seasoning blend

- ½ tsp salt

- ¼ tsp pepper

- ½ cup Parmesan cheese (finely grated)

- ½ cup whole fat milk

- 1 lb ground beef

- 1 lb ground pork sausage

Directions:

1. Line a big cookie sheet with foil and put it away. In a bowl, mix the milk with the Parmesan cheese. Let it sit for about 5 minutes, then stir. In a big bowl, mix together both meats, the spices, and the egg.

2. Add the cheese that has been soaked to the meats. When you use your hands, gently mix everything until it is well mixed. Be careful not to work too much.

3. You can use an ice cream scoop to scoop the meat mixture into your hands and roll it into balls. When all of the meat mixture has been used, put the balls on the foil-lined cookie sheet. Take a cookie sheet and put it in the oven. Turn on the broiler. For about 8 minutes, broil the meatballs until they are brown and crispy. Then carefully flip them over and broil for another 4 minutes.

4. Make sure your oven is at 400°F. Keep the meatballs in the range for another 10 minutes, or until they're cooked through. Remove them from the oven and let them cool down to room temperature before eating them.

5. Clean parchment paper should move the meatballs to a clean cookie sheet. It will take about 3 hours, or until they are set and rigid.

6. Meatballs can be stored in the freezer for up to four months. Transfer them to a bag or container and put them back in the freezer for that long. To heat them up, put them in the microwave or oven for a few minutes.

Easy Slow Cooker Keto Carnivore Beef Stew

Ingredients:

- 8 ounce mushrooms quartered

- 2 cups cauliflower chopped

- 1 large carrot chopped

- 1 large onion chopped

- 4 cloves garlic minced

- 2 tsp dried thyme

- 2 tsp salt

- 2 pounds beef marrow bones

- 2 pounds chuck roast cubed

- 2 tbsp beef tallow or other cooking oil

- 6 cups b2 broth

- 1 tsp ground black pepper

Directions:

1. Turn the slow cooker on low and place the marrow bones in the center of the insert.
2. Cube the roast. Heat tallow in a large skillet over high heat. Arrange the meat in a single layer and sear evenly on all sides. Cook in batches if needed. Once cooked, add to the pot.
3. Rinse and chop all vegetables. Gather the herbs. Place everything all in the pot on top of the meat.
4. Pour broth over it all. Season with salt and pepper.
5. Cover and cook on low for 6-8 hours.

Keto Breakfast Casserol

Ingredients:

- 1 cup cheddar cheese shredded

- ¼ cup Parmesan shredded

- ½ teaspoon dried thyme

- ½ teaspoon salt

- ½ teaspoon ground black pepper

- 1 tablespoon grass-fed butter

- 1 medium onion diced

- 2 cloves garlic minced

- 1 pound chicken sausage

- 10 whole eggs

Directions:

1. Preheat the oven to 350°F (175°C).

2. Warm butter in a frying pan over medium heat. Sauté the onion and garlic together for 5 minutes.

3. Remove the sausage from its casing and add to the pan also.

4. Break apart into smaller pieces and brown all sides evenly, about 8 minutes.

5. While the sausage browns, whisk 10 eggs in a large bowl.

6. Mix in the cheese, thyme, salt, and pepper.

7. Transfer meat to an 8×8-inch (20×20 cm) glass baking or casserole dish. Arrange in a single, even layer on the bottom.

8. Pour the egg mixture over the meat.

9. Gently jiggle or tap the dish so the egg can settle down around the meat.

10. Bake for 20 minutes, until eggs are set and top is golden brown. Let rest 5 minutes before slicing and serving warm.

Low-Carb Breakfast Lasagna

Ingredients:

- 1/2 cup coconut cream or dairy cream

- 3/4 cup bone broth

- 1 medium zucchini 3/4 of a pound

- 2 cups mozzarella cheese shredded

- 9 whole eggs

- 1 tablespoon salt

- 1 teaspoon ground black pepper

- 1 pound chicken sausage

Directions:

1. Preheat the oven to 350 degrees F.

2. Whisk the eggs with salt and pepper. Warm a bit of butter or coconut oil in a skillet and scramble the eggs. Remove from heat and set aside.

3. In the same skillet, brown the sausage. Once it is cooked, add the cream and broth to the pan.

4. Simmer together with the sausage for 5 to 10 minutes, until the liquid reduces a bit.

5. Spiralize or julienne the zucchini, go for long, broad pieces.

6. In an 8 by 8-inch baking dish, spoon a layer of sausage and liquid to the bottom of the dish.

7. Arrange 1 the slices of zucchini across in one direction.

8. Divide the scrambled eggs in 1 and spread over the first layer of zucchini. Top this layer with 1 cup shredded cheese.

9. Repeat the layers again. Sausage with creamy broth, zucchini, egg and cheese.

10. Press down on the layers to flatten.

11. My dish was almost overflowing but the volume greatly reduces as the lasagna bakes.

12. Bake for 40 minutes until the cheese is golden and bubbly.

13. Slice and serve warm. Save leftovers in the fridge. Its great cold! I had a cold slice for lunch the next day.

Cheddar Cheese Sauce On Turkey

Ingredients:

- 2 tbsp butter + more to grease

- pepper to taste 1 cup milk or 1 & 1

- 1 cup shredded cheddar cheese, salt to taste

- 4 slices (1 ounce each) (1 ounce each) turkey breast, cooked

Directions:

1. Grease a small square baking dish (about 6x6 inches) with a little butter.
2. In the dish, arrange the turkey pieces.
3. Over medium heat, place a saucepan. Melt the butter in the pan.
4. Simmer for a few minutes with the turkey, salt, pepper, and 1-and-1.

5. Cook until the cheese has melted and is thoroughly combined with the other Ingredients:.

6. Turn the heat off.

7. Pour the sauce over the turkey.

8. Preheat the oven to 350°F and bake for 20 minutes, or until the sauce is boiling.

Comfit Duck Legs

Ingredients:

- a quarter teaspoon of kosher salt

- to taste freshly ground pepper

- 2 cups fat de canard (that was retained)

- 3-4 teaspoon peppercorns, whole

- 2 duck legs with the thigh shaved of extra fat and kept

- butter (3-5 tablespoons)

- to taste table salt

Directions:

1. Place the duck legs with the skin side down on a big platter. Season with kosher salt and freshly ground black pepper.

2. In a baking dish, pour the duck fat.

3. Refrigerate the duck legs for 10 to 12 hours after stacking them in the baking dish.

4. Remove the duck from the water and rinse it in cold water. Remove the salt and pepper with a soft cloth.

5. Using paper towels, pat dry.

6. Remove the duck fat and set it in a cast-iron enameled kettle.

7. Sprinkle peppercorns on top of the fat. Season it with salt.

8. Place the duck in the pot with the skin side down. On top of the duck, spread some duck grease. Place in a warm oven, covered.

9. Bake for approximately 2-3 hours at 350 degrees F, or until the flesh comes away from the b2.

10. Into a basin, drain the fat from the casserole. Keep the fat for storing meat or using in another dish.

11. If you want to serve the duck legs straight immediately, place them on a pan with the skin side down.

12. Sear the skin until it is crisp and golden in the pan over medium high heat.

13. Remove the meat off the b2s and store it in a ceramic container if you wish to consume it after a few days.

14. Pour some of the grease that has remained over the meat. (Fat should cover the meat by at least a quarter inch.) Refrigerate the container until ready to use. It might last a month.

Crispy Thighs Of Chicken

Ingredients:

- 2 tablespoons melted butter or lard

- to taste freshly ground pepper

- to taste kosher salt

- 6 skinless chicken thighs

Directions:

1. Using paper towels, pat the chicken dry. Salt & pepper to taste.

2. Toss thoroughly.

3. Place the chicken pieces in a single layer on a baking sheet with the skin side up. Drizzle some butter on top.

4. Roast for 20–30 minutes or until cooked through in a preheated oven at 400° F. The temperature in the thickest section of the meat should be 165 degrees Fahrenheit.

5. Broil for a few minutes if you want the skin to be crisp.

Strip Steak

Ingredients:

- 2(8-ounce) strip steaks

- 2 teaspoons kosher salt

Directions:

1. Pat dry each steak and rub the salt over each side.

2. 30 minutes before cooking the steaks, let them cool down in the fridge.

3. Heat a cast-iron pan on a high flame.

4. To hold the steaks, use tongs to sear the fat strip that runs down 2 side for 3 minutes. A 12-inch-thick piece of fat should be roasted for another minute. Place the steaks in the pan and cook them for 4 minutes, or until they are d2.

5. Turn the steaks over and cook them for another 4 minutes, or until the meat is d2.

6. There are four ways to check the steaks for d2ness: at 125°F for rare, 135°F for medium-rare, 145°F for medium, and 155°F for medium-well.

7. To cut the steaks, move them to a cutting board, cover them loosely with aluminum foil, and let them rest for 10 minutes before cutting them.

8. Slice the steaks and serve. TIP: This steak is already tasty, but you can add black pepper and other spices if you want more flavor. If you add more fat to your meal, add butter to the steak as it is resting.

B2-In Rib Eye

Ingredients:

- 2 (1-pound) b2-in rib-eye steaks

- 2 teaspoons kosher salt

Directions:

1. Make sure to rub salt on both sides of the steaks. Then, take a 30 minute break.

2. Over high heat, put a giant, cast-iron pan on. Place the steaks in the pan and cook them for five minutes without moving them.

3. Turn the steaks over, cook them for another 4 minutes to get them medium-rare, and then serve them immediately.

4. Make sure the inside temperature is 125°F for rare, 135°F for medium, 145°F for medium-medium, and 155°F for well d2.

5. To cut the steaks, move them to a cutting board, cover them loosely with aluminum foil,

and let them rest for 10 minutes before cutting them.

6. Add 1 teaspoon of minced garlic and 1 teaspoon of paprika to your food if you want to spice it up a little bit.

Roasted B2 Marrow

Ingredients:

- 1 tablespoon kosher salt

- 2 pounds marrow b2s

- 2 cups water

Directions:

1. Preheat the oven to 450°F.
2. Mix the water and salt until the salt is thoroughly mixed in a large bowl.
3. Salty water should be used to clean the b2s. Gently rub the b2s to get rid of the salt.
4. A paper towel can be used to pat the b2s dry.
5. Then, put them in a roasting pan. If the b2s are cut in 1, stand them up.
6. If they are cut in 1 lengthwise, put them in the pan marrow-side up.

7. Roast for about 20 minutes, or until the food is d2. Serve right away.

Fish Cakes With Aioli Recipe

Ingredients:

- Chili powder, 1 tablespoon

- Olive oil, 2 cup

- Fish, 2 pound

- Cilantro, 2 tablespoon

- Mayonnaise, 2 cup

- Avocado, 3 slices

- Salt to taste

- Fish cake, 2 pound

- Aioli sauce, 2 cup

- Orange juice, 2 tablespoon

- Garlic powder, 2 cup

- Pepper to taste

Directions:

1. Wash the fish and let it dry.
2. Take a small bowl.
3. Add the fish into it.
4. Add the orange juice, garlic powder and lemon juice.
5. Add the chili powder and pepper.
6. Then add the cilantro and mix them all well.
7. Marinate your fish for some time.
8. After marinating, cook the fish in a pan for few minutes.
9. You can add salt and pepper as required.
10. Serve it with aioli sauce and mayonnaise.

Salmon And Cream Cheese Bites Recipe

Ingredients:

- Cilantro, 2 tablespoon

- Mayonnaise, 2 cup

- Avocado, 3 slices

- Salt to taste

- Pepper to taste

- Salmon, 2 pound

- Cream cheese, 3 cups

- Garlic powder, 2 cup

- Chili powder, 1 tablespoon

- Olive oil, 2 cup

Directions:

1. Take a small bowl.

2. Add the fish into it.

3. Add the orange juice, garlic powder and lemon juice.

4. Add the chili powder and pepper.

5. Then add the cilantro and mix them all well.

6. Marinate your fish for some time.

7. After marinating, cook the fish in a pan for few minutes.

8. Make small pieces of your cooked fish.

9. Serve it with avocado slices and cheese.

Sashimi Rolls Recipe

Ingredients:

- Fish, 2 pound

- Cilantro, 2 tablespoon

- Mayonnaise, 2 cup

- Avocado, 3 slices

- Wonton wrappers, as required

- Salt to taste

- Sashimi, 2 pound

- Garlic powder, 2 cup

- Chili powder, 1 tablespoon

- Olive oil, 2 cup

- Pepper to taste

Directions:

1. Wash your salmon fish and let it dry.

2. Add salmon fish into it.

3. Add in the spices.

4. Then add cilantro and mix them all well.

5. Marinate your fish for some time.

6. After marinating, cook the fish in a pan for few minutes.

7. Make rolls of it in wonton wrappers.

8. Your dish is ready to be served.

Crispy Chicken Thighs

Ingredients:

- 2 tbsps salt

- 2 sprigs fresh rosemary, chopped

- 12 chicken thighs

- 4 tbsps olive oil

Directions:

1. Preheat oven to 450° F.
2. Rub salt on each chicken thigh and place on a greased baking tray.
3. Drizzle the olive oil over the chicken thighs and top with the rosemary.
4. Bake for 40 minutes until golden and crispy. Enjoy!

Roasted Paprica Turkey Wings

Ingredients:

- 1 tbs olive oil

- Salt and pepper, to taste

- 1 tsp paprika

- 15 lb turkey wings

Directions:

1. Preheat the oven to 375° F.
2. Line a baking pan with foil, and place a metal rack on top.
3. Remove the wingtips and any excess fat or skin.
4. Place the wings on the rack and drizzle with olive oil, then season with salt and pepper.

5. Roast until the wings are cooked, about 40 minutes.
6. During the last five minutes of cooking, sprinkle paprika over the wings and return to the oven.

Baked Chicken Thighs

Ingredients:

- 2 teaspoons dried oregano

- 1 teaspoon dried thyme

- Salt and freshly ground black pepper, to taste

- 1½ pounds b2-in chicken thighs

- 2 tablespoons butter, divided

- 1 tablespoon fresh lemon juice

- 1 tablespoon lemon zest, grated

Directions:

1. Preheat the oven to 420 degrees F.
2. In a large mixing bowl, add 1 tablespoon of the butter, lemon juice, lemon zest, dried herbs, salt, and black pepper and mix well.

3. Add the chicken thighs and coat with the mixture generously.
4. Refrigerate to marinate for at least 20 minutes.
5. In an oven-proof skillet, melt the remaining butter over medium-high heat and sear the chicken thighs for about 2-3 minutes per side.
6. Remove from the heat and immediately transfer the skillet into the oven.
7. Bake for about 10 minutes.
8. Remove from the oven and set aside for about 2-3 minutes.
9. Serve hot.

Grilled Duck Breast

Ingredients:

- 2 tablespoons fresh thyme, chopped

- Salt and freshly ground black pepper, to taste

- 2 duck breasts

- 2 shallots, sliced thinly

- 1 tablespoon fresh ginger, minced

Directions:

1. In a large bowl, place the shallots, ginger, thyme, salt and black pepper and mix well.
2. Add the duck breasts and coat with marinade evenly.
3. Refrigerate to marinate for about 2–12 hours.
4. Preheat the grill to medium-high heat. Grease the grill grate.

5. Place the duck breast onto the grill, skin-side down, and cook for about 6–8 minutes per side.
6. Serve hot.

Easy Grilled Shrimp

Ingredients:

- 1 teaspoon seafood seasoning

- ¼ teaspoon white sugar

- ⅛ teaspoon cayenne pepper

- Salt to taste

- 2 tablespoons extra-virgin olive oil

- ½ lemon, juiced

- 1 pound shrimp, shelled and deveined

Directions:

1. Combine olive oil, lemon juice, seafood seasoning, sugar, cayenne, and salt in a small bowl; stir until marinade is well mixed.

2. Thread shrimp on metal skewers and pat dry.

3. Brush with marinade and refrigerate.

4. Preheat an outdoor grill for medium-high heat and lightly oil the grate.

5. Cook shrimp on the hot grill until the edges begin to turn white, 1 to 2 minutes.

6. Turn and continue grilling until shrimp is white and no longer translucent, 1 to 2 minutes longer. Serve warm.

Steamed Tuna Fish

Ingredients:

- ½ cup minced fresh ginger root

- 3 cloves garlic, minced

- 1 teaspoon salt

- 1 teaspoon ground black pepper

- 2 pounds fresh tuna steaks

- ½ cup soy sauce

- ½ cup sherry

- ½ cup vegetable oil

- 1 bunch green onions, finely chopped

Directions:

1. Place tuna steaks in a steamer over 1 inch of boiling water, and cover.

118

2. Cook 6 to 8 minutes, or until fish flakes easily with a fork.
3. Meanwhile, in a medium saucepan, combine soy sauce, sherry, vegetable oil, green onions, ginger, garlic, salt, and black pepper. Bring to a boil.
4. Remove tuna steaks from steamer, and place in a serving dish.
5. Pour sauce over tuna steaks, and serve immediately.

Marinated Flank Steak

Ingredients:

- 1 tbsp olive oil

- 1 lime

- 1 lb flank steak

- ½ cup salsa

- 1 clove garlic (minced)

Directions:

1. Put the salsa, garlic, olive oil, and lime juice in a zip top bag. Shake the Ingredients: in the bag to mix everything thoroughly.

2. Add the flank steak to the mixture in the bag. Re-seal the bag after letting out as much air as possible. Let the steak marinade in the fridge for at least 4 hours.

3. When it is time to cook the steak, remove it from the zip top bag, and discard the marinade.
4. Grill or broil the flank steak to your preference (medium, rare, well-d2, etc.); however, keep in mind that flank steak can become extremely tough if it is overcooked.
5. Let it rest for about 10 minutes, and then slice the meat against the grain into thin slices. Serve immediately.

Freezer Breakfast Sandwiches

Ingredients:

- 8 x 1 oz slices Swiss cheese

- 3 oz buffalo chicken

- 3 oz roast beef

- 8 large eggs

- 1 tsp sea salt

- 1 tsp ground black pepper

- 8 keto-friendly buns

Directions:

1. Preheat the oven to 350°F.
2. Spray a muffin tin with cooking spray and crack an egg into each of 8 cups.
3. Season with sea salt and ground black pepper.

4. Bake for 10-15 minutes depending on your preference.

5. In the meantime, prepare 8 sandwich-size freezer bags, placing a keto-friendly bun (cut open) on each piece.

6. Add ¾ oz meat to each sandwich; 1 chicken and 1 beef.

7. Add a slice of Swiss cheese to each sandwich.

8. When the eggs are d2, remove them from the oven and let them cool for 2-4 minutes.

9. Scoop 2 egg onto each sandwich and prepare it for the freezer.

10. When you are ready to eat them, remove them from the freezer and heat it in the microwave for a few minutes.

Carnivore Beef Broth

Ingredients:

- 2 tbsp organic apple cider vinegar

- 1 tsp sea salt (to taste)

- 12 garlic cloves

- 2 lb grass-fed marrow b2s

- 1 gallon filtered water

Directions:

1. Brown the marrow b2s in a pan that has been sprayed with cooking spray.

2. This will give the food a little extra taste. Add everything to a Crockpot.

3. Cook it on high until the broth starts to boil, then turn it down to low and cook for another 10-24 hours.

4. Remember that the longer the broth, the better.
5. Let the broth cool down, then put it in your own glass jars or other containers.
6. Then, put it in the fridge for a few days or in the freezer for longer.

Carnivore Steak Nuggets

Ingredients:

- ½ tsp homemade seas2d salt Dip (optional)

- ¼ cup mayonnaise

- ¼ cup sour cream (organic, cultured)

- 1+ tsp chipotle paste to taste

- ½ tsp homemade ranch dressing and dip mix

- ¼ medium lime (juiced)

- 1 lb venison or beef steak cut into chunks

- 1 large egg

- Lard or palm oil Breading

- ½ cup grated Parmesan cheese

- ½ cup pork panko

Directions:

1. For the dip, put all the Ingredients: together and mix them well. 1 tbsp of the chipotle paste makes a medium-spice variety.

2. Depending on how spicy you like, you can use more or less.

3. Keep it in the fridge for 30 minutes before eating it, and remember that it can be kept in the refrigerator for up to a week.

4. Prepare: Mix the pork panko with Parmesan cheese and seasoning salt, then set it apart to cool down.

5. Place the beaten egg in 2 bowl and the breading mix in another.

6. Mix them together and put them in a pan.

7. Dip the steak into the egg, then bread it.

8. You can put it on a wax paper-lined pan or plate.

9. They should be frozen for 30 minutes before they are fried.

10. This way, the breading won't come away from the meat when it's fried, so it will stay together.

11. Lard or cooking oil should be at 325°F.

12. Fry the frozen steak nuggets until they're brown, about 2-3 minutes, then remove them from the pan.

13. When you're d2, put it on a paper towel-lined dish, add a little salt, and serve it with or without a dip.

Freezer Breakfast Sandwiches

Ingredients:

- 8 x 1 oz slices Swiss cheese

- 3 oz buffalo chicken

- 3 oz roast beef

- 8 large eggs

- 1 tsp sea salt

- 1 tsp ground black pepper

- 8 keto-friendly buns

Directions:

1. The oven should be set to 350°F.
2. When making muffins, spray a muffin pan with cooking spray.
3. Crack an egg into each of the 8 cups. Then, add sea salt and ground black pepper. Bake

for 10-15 minutes, depending on how long you want it to cook.

4. In the meantime, make 8 sandwich-sized freezer bags by putting a keto-friendly bun (cut open) on each piece.

5. Do this while you wait. Add 34 oz of meat to each sandwich; 1 chicken and 1 beef.

6. Make sure there is enough meat on each sandwich. The Swiss cheese should go on each sandwich.

7. Eggs should be out of the oven when they're d2. Let them cool down for about 2 to 4 minutes before eating them. Each sandwich should have 2 egg and be ready to be put in the fridge.

8. Make sure you take them out of the freezer when ready to eat.

9. Heat them in the microwave for a few minutes.

Three Cheese Omelette

Ingredients:

- 1/2 ounce Gruyere shredded

- 1/2 ounce cheddar shredded

- 1/4 teaspoon salt

- 1/4 teaspoon ground black pepper

- 1/2 tablespoon grass-fed butter

- 3 whole eggs whisked

- 1/2 ounce Gouda shredded

Directions:

1. Warm the butter over medium heat in a skillet.
2. Once the pan is warm, pour the eggs in.
3. Arrange the cheese down the center of the omelette. Wait until the eggs are cooked,

then use a spatula to fold in the sides, so the omelette is folded in thirds.

4. Serve warm with a salt and pepper on top.

No Bake Keto Cheesecake

Ingredients:

- 1½ tablespoons heavy whipping cream

- ½ tablespoons powdered Monkfruit Sweetener

- ⅛ teaspoon vanilla extract

- 2 ounces cream cheese room temperature

- 1 tablespoon sour cream

Directions:

1. Beat all Ingredients: together with an electric mixer. Continue mixing until smooth.
2. Serve immediately or chill for 30-60 minutes.

Soup With Creamy Chicken.

Ingredients:

- 4 cup b2 broth from chicken

- to taste salt

- to taste pepper

- 4 cups shredded cooked chicken breast

- 1 a gallon of heavy cream

- 4 tbsp. melted butter

- 8 oz. cubed cream cheese

Directions:

1. Place a medium saucepan over medium heat. Melt the butter in the pan. Add the chicken and cook for a few minutes, or until it is nicely coated with butter.

2. Mix in the cream cheese well.

3. Stir in the broth and cream after the cream cheese has melted.

4. Stir in the salt and pepper.

5. Serve immediately in soup bowls.

Tomato And Basil Meatballs

Ingredients:

- 2 small celery stalks, finely chopped

- 2 garlic cloves, minced

- 4 large tomatoes, seeded and roughly chopped

- 4 leaves fresh basil, finely chopped

- 1 teaspoon kosher salt

- 1 teaspoon freshly ground black pepper

- 1 teaspoon paprika

- ½ cup tomato sauce

- 1 tablespoon tomato paste

- 1 egg

- ¼ cup grated Parmesan cheese

- 1 pound 80/20 ground chuck beef

- 1 tablespoon Italian Spice Blend

- 2 tablespoons olive oil

- ½ small onion, finely chopped

- ¾ cup beef broth or chicken broth

Directions:

1. The oven should be set to 400°F.

2. A baking sheet should be lined with parchment paper or a silic2 mat to not stick to the pan. Cover a piece of food with a paper towel.

3. A large bowl is the best place to put the egg, Parmesan, ground beef, and Italian seasoning blend. With your hands, mix them.

4. Do this step with your hands instead of a spoon.

5. Making meatballs with your hands, divide the mixture into eight equal parts.

6. Put them on the baking sheet and bake for 20 minutes when they are d2 .

7. Then, move the meatballs to a plate that has been lined with paper towels.

8. In a 2-quart saucepan, heat the olive oil on medium-low heat until it starts to smoke. Turn down the heat to low.

9. Add the onions, celery, and garlic, and cook them for about 5 minutes.

10. It's time to put in the tomatoes and basil, as well as salt and pepper, and stir until they are all mixed.

11. They should be gently stirred to make sure they are covered in the sauce.

12. Cover and cook for an hour. Serve right away.

Braised Oxtail

Ingredients:

- ¾ cup beef broth

- 1 tablespoon tomato paste

- 1 teaspoon kosher salt

- 1 teaspoon freshly ground black pepper

- 1 teaspoon garlic powder

- 1 teaspoon paprika

- 3 tablespoons olive oil

- 2 pounds oxtails

- ½ onion, thinly sliced

- 2 celery stalks, chopped

- 1 carrot, chopped

- ½ teaspoon ground ginger

Directions:

1. Preheat the oven to 300°F.

2. Heat the oil in a nonstick pan, heat it over medium-high heat.

3. Add the oxtails and cook them for about 4 or 5 minutes on each side until they are brown on all sides.

4. They will be put in a baking dish and put away.

5. This is how it works: Add the onions and celery to a pan and cook them over low heat for 5 minutes. Stir often to make sure the vegetables don't burn.

6. While the vegetables are cooking, make the oxtail.

7. Add the beef broth, tomato paste, salt, pepper, garlic powder, paprika, and ginger to the baking dish with the oxtail. Bake for an hour and a 1.

8. Add the vegetables to the baking dish and stir them until they are all mixed. Bake for 3 hours. Serve it hot.

Carnivore Diet Bone Broth Recipe

Ingredients:

- 6 pounds beef b2 s

- ¼ cup raw apple cider vinegar optional

Directions:

1. Arrange the bones in a single layer in a large roasting tray and place them in the oven at 450°F (232°C) for about 20 minutes, until golden brown. NOTE: This step is optional and followed to affect the end flavor of the broth.

2. Place all the bones in a large stockpot. Fill with enough water to fully cover the material.

3. Pour in optional vinegar.

4. Bring the water to a boil, then reduce down to a simmer. Adjust the flame and pot lid to maintain a low simmer.

5. Cook for at least 18 hours, and up to 72 hours.

6. I tend to pull my batch after about 24 hours.

7. Check periodically to ensure the water remains over the b2 s. Add extra water as needed.

8. Let the broth cool slightly. If a layer of scum or film appears over the top, skim it off with a slotted spoon.

9. Strain the broth through a fine-mesh strainer or cheesecloth.

10. Store in glass jars in the fridge for up to 5 days or in the freezer for longer.

www.ingramcontent.com/pod-product-compliance
Lightning Source LLC
Chambersburg PA
CBHW060234030426
42335CB00014B/1457